My Mediterranean Dash Diet Recipe Book

Recipe Book

A Collection of Delicious Mediterranean Dash Diet Recipes for Your Daily Meals

Kathyrn Solano

By reading this document, the reader agrees that under no circumstances is the author responsible for any losses, direct or indirect, which are incurred as a result of the use of information contained within this document, including, but not limited to, — errors, omissions, or inaccuracies.

Table of contents

SNACKS RECIPES

Chunky Monkey Trail Mix

Servings: 6

Cooking Time: 1 Hour 30 Minutes

Ingredients:

1 cup cashews, halved

2 cups raw walnuts, chopped or halved

⅓ cup coconut sugar

1 cup coconut flakes, unsweetened and make sure you have big flakes and not shredded

6 ounces dried banana slices

1 ½ teaspoons coconut oil at room temperature

1 teaspoon vanilla extract

½ cup of chocolate chips

Directions:

Turn your crockpot to high and add the cashews, walnuts, vanilla, coconut oil, and sugar. Combine until the ingredients are well mixed and then cook for 45 minutes.

Reduce the temperature on your crockpot to low.

Continue to cook the mixture for another 20 minutes.

Place a piece of parchment paper on your counter.

Once the mix is done cooking, remove it from the crockpot and set on top of the parchment paper.

Let the mixture sit and cool for 20 minutes.

Pour the contents into a bowl and add the dried bananas and chocolate chips. Gently mix the ingredients together. You can store the mixture in Ziplock bags for a quick and easy snack.

Nutrition Info: calories: 250, fats: 6 grams, carbohydrates: 1grams, protein: 4 grams

Fig-pecan Energy Bites

Servings: 6

Cooking Time: 20 Minutes

Ingredients:

½ cup chopped pecans

2 tablespoons honey

¾ cup dried figs, about 6 to 8, diced

2 tablespoons wheat flaxseed

¼ cup quick oats

2 tablespoons regular or powdered peanut butter

Directions:

Combine the figs, quick oats, pecans, peanut butter, and flaxseed into a bowl. Stir the ingredients well.

Drizzle honey onto the ingredients and mix everything with a wooden spoon. Do your best to press all the ingredients into the honey as you are stirring. If you start to struggle because the mixture is too sticky, set it in the freezer for 3 to 5 minutes.

Divide the mixture into four sections.

Take a wet rag and get your hands damp. You don't want them too wet or they won't work well with the mixture.

Divide each of the four sections into 3 separate sections.

Take one of the three sections and roll them up. Repeat with each section so you have a dozen energy bites once you are done.

If you want to firm them up, you can place them into the freezer for a few minutes. Otherwise, you can enjoy them as soon as they are little energy balls.

To store them, you'll want to keep them in a sealed container and set them in the fridge. They can be stored for about a week.

Nutrition Info: calories: 157, fats: 6 grams, carbohydrates: 26 grams, protein: 3 grams.

Baked Apples Mediterranean Style

Servings: 4

Cooking Time: 25 Minutes

Ingredients:

½ lemon, squeezed for juice

1 ½ pounds of peeled and sliced apples

¼ teaspoon cinnamon

Directions:

Set the temperature of your oven to 350 degrees Fahrenheit so it can preheat.

Take a piece of parchment paper and lay on top of a baking pan.

Combine your lemon juice, cinnamon, and apples into a medium bowl and mix well.

Pour the apples onto the baking pan and arrange them so they are not doubled up.

Place the pan in the oven and set your timer to 2minutes. The apples should be tender but not mushy.

Remove from the oven, plate and enjoy!

Nutrition Info: calories: 90, fats: 0.3 grams, carbohydrates: 24 grams, protein: 0.5 grams.

Strawberry Popsicle

Servings: 5

Cooking Time: 10 Minutes

Ingredients:

½ cup almond milk

1 ½ cups fresh strawberries

Directions:

Using a blender or hand mixer, combine the almond milk and strawberries thoroughly in a bowl.

Using popsicle molds, pour the mixture into the molds and place the sticks into the mixture.

Set in the freezer for at least 4 hours.

Serve and enjoy—especially on a hot day!

Nutritional information: calories: 3 fats: 0.5 grams, carbohydrates: 7 grams, protein: 0.6 grams.

Frozen Blueberry Yogurt

Servings: 6

Cooking Time: 30 Minutes

Ingredients:

⅔ cup honey

2 cups chilled yogurt

1 pint fresh blueberries

1 juiced and zested lime or lemon. You can even substitute an orange if your tastes prefer.

Directions:

With a saucepan on your burner set to medium heat, add the honey, juiced fruit, zest, and blueberries.

Stir the mixture continuously as it begins to simmer for 15 minutes.

When the liquid is nearly gone, pour the contents into a bowl and place in the fridge for several minutes. You will want to stir the ingredients and check to see if they are chilled.

Once the fruit is chilled, combine with the yogurt.

Mix until the ingredients are well incorporated and enjoy.

Nutrition Info: calories: 233, fats: 3 grams, carbohydrates: 52 grams, protein: 3.5 grams.

LUNCH AND DINNER RECIPES

Marinated Tuna Steak

Servings: 4

Cooking Time: 15-20 Minute

Ingredients:

Olive oil (2 tbsp.)

Orange juice (.25 cup)

Soy sauce (.25 cup)

Lemon juice (1 tbsp.)

Fresh parsley (2 tbsp.)

Garlic clove (1)

Ground black pepper (.5 tsp.)

Fresh oregano (.5 tsp.)

Tuna steaks (4 - 4 oz. Steaks)

Directions:

Mince the garlic and chop the oregano and parsley.

In a glass container, mix the pepper, oregano, garlic, parsley, lemon juice, soy sauce, olive oil, and orange juice.

Warm the grill using the high heat setting. Grease the grate with oil.

Add to tuna steaks and cook for five to six minutes. Turn and baste with the marinated sauce.

Cook another five minutes or until it's the way you like it. Discard the remaining marinade.

Nutrition Info: Calories: 200;Protein: 27.4 grams; Fat: 7.9 grams

Garlic And Shrimp Pasta

Servings: 4

Cooking Time: 15 Minutes

Ingredients:

6 ounces whole wheat spaghetti

12 ounces raw shrimp, peeled and deveined, cut into 1-inch pieces

1 bunch asparagus, trimmed

1 large bell pepper, thinly sliced

1 cup fresh peas

3 garlic cloves, chopped

1 and ¼ teaspoons kosher salt

½ and ½ cups non-fat plain yogurt

3 tablespoon lemon juice

1 tablespoon extra-virgin olive oil

½ teaspoon fresh ground black pepper

¼ cup pine nuts, toasted

Directions:

Take a large sized pot and bring water to a boil

Add your spaghetti and cook them for about minutes less than the directed package instruction

Add shrimp, bell pepper, asparagus and cook for about 2- 4 minutes until the shrimp are tender

Drain the pasta and the contents well

Take a large bowl and mash garlic until a paste form

Whisk in yogurt, parsley, oil, pepper and lemon juice into the garlic paste

Add pasta mix and toss well

Serve by sprinkling some pine nuts!

Enjoy!

Meal Prep/Storage Options: Store in airtight containers in your fridge for 1-3 days.

Nutrition Info: Calories: 406;Fat: 22g;Carbohydrates: 28g;Protein: 26g

Paprika Butter Shrimps

Servings: 2

Cooking Time: 30 Minutes

Ingredients:

¼ tablespoon smoked paprika

1/8 cup sour cream

½ pound tiger shrimps

1/8 cup butter

Salt and black pepper, to taste

Directions:

Preheat the oven to 390 degrees F and grease a baking dish.

Mix together all the ingredients in a large bowl and transfer into the baking dish.

Place in the oven and bake for about 15 minutes.

Place paprika shrimp in a dish and set aside to cool for meal prepping. Divide it in 2 containers and cover the lid. Refrigerate for 1-2 days and reheat in microwave before serving.

Nutrition Info: Calories: 330; Carbohydrates: 1.; Protein: 32.6g; Fat: 21.5g; Sugar: 0.2g; Sodium: 458mg

Mediterranean Avocado Salmon Salad

Servings: 4

Cooking Time: 10 Minutes

Ingredients:

1 lb skinless salmon fillets

Marinade/Dressing:

3 tbsp olive oil

2 tbsp lemon juice fresh, squeezed

1 tbsp red wine vinegar, optional

1 tbsp fresh chopped parsley

2 tsp garlic minced

1 tsp dried oregano

1 tsp salt

Cracked pepper, to taste

Salad:

4 cups Romaine (or Cos) lettuce leaves, washed and dried

1 large cucumber, diced

2 Roma tomatoes, diced

1 red onion, sliced

1 avocado, sliced

1/2 cup feta cheese crumbled

1/3 cup pitted Kalamata olives or black olives, sliced

Lemon wedges to serve

Directions:

In a jug, whisk together the olive oil, lemon juice, red wine vinegar, chopped parsley, garlic minced, oregano, salt and pepper

Pour out half of the marinade into a large, shallow dish, refrigerate the remaining marinade to use as the dressing

Coat the salmon in the rest of the marinade

Place a skillet pan or grill over medium-high, add 1 tbsp oil and sear salmon on both sides until crispy and cooked through

Allow the salmon to cool

Distribute the salmon among the containers, store in the fridge for 2-3 days

To Serve: Prepare the salad by placing the romaine lettuce, cucumber, roma tomatoes, red onion, avocado, feta cheese, and olives in a large salad bowl. Reheat the salmon in the microwave for 30seconds to 1 minute or until heated through.

Slice the salmon and arrange over salad. Drizzle the salad with the remaining untouched dressing, serve with lemon wedges.

Nutrition Info: Calories:411; Carbs: 12g; Total Fat: 27g; Protein: 28g

Beet Kale Salad

Servings: 6

Cooking Time: 50 Minutes

Ingredients:

1 bunch of kale, washed and dried, ribs removed, chopped

6 pieces washed beets, peeled and dried and cut into ½ inches

½ teaspoon dried rosemary

½ teaspoon garlic powder

salt

pepper

olive oil

¼ medium red onion, thinly sliced

1-2 tablespoons slivered almonds, toasted

¼ cup olive oil

Juice of 1½ lemon

¼ cup honey

¼ teaspoon garlic powder

1 teaspoon dried rosemary

salt

pepper

Directions:

Preheat oven to 400 degrees F.

Take a bowl and toss the kale with some salt, pepper, and olive oil.

Lightly oil a baking sheet and add the kale.

Roast in the oven for 5 minutes, and then remove and place to the side.

Place beets in a bowl and sprinkle with a bit of rosemary, garlic powder, pepper, and salt; ensure beets are coated well.

Spread the beets on the oiled baking sheet, place on the middle rack of your oven, and roast for 45 minutes, turning twice.

Make the lemon vinaigrette by whisking all of the listed Ingredients: in a bowl.

Once the beets are ready, remove from the oven and allow it to cool.

Take a medium-sized salad bowl and add kale, onions, and beets.

Dress with lemon honey vinaigrette and toss well.

Garnish with toasted almonds.

Enjoy!

Nutrition Info: Calories: 245, Total Fat: 17.6 g, Saturated Fat: 2.6 g, Cholesterol: 0 mg, Sodium: 77 mg, Total Carbohydrate: 22.9 g, Dietary Fiber: 3 g, Total Sugars: 17.7 g, Protein: 2.4 g, Vitamin D: 0 mcg, Calcium: 50 mg, Iron: 1 mg, Potassium: 416 mg

Moroccan Fish

Servings: 12

Cooking Time: 1 Hour 25 Minutes

Ingredients:

Garbanzo beans (15 oz. Can)

Red bell peppers (2)

Large carrot (1)

Vegetable oil (1 tbsp.)

Onion (1)

Garlic (1 clove)

Tomatoes (3 chopped/14.5 oz can)

Olives (4 chopped)

Chopped fresh parsley (.25 cup)

Ground cumin (.25 cup)

Paprika (3 tbsp.)

Chicken bouillon granules (2 tbsp.)

Cayenne pepper (1 tsp.)

Salt (to your liking)

Tilapia fillets (5 lb.)

Directions:

Drain and rinse the beans. Thinly slice the carrot and onion. Mince the garlic and chop the olives. Discard the seeds from the peppers and slice them into strips.

Warm the oil in a frying pan using the medium temperature setting. Toss in the onion and garlic. Simmer them for approximately five minutes.

Fold in the bell peppers, beans, tomatoes, carrots, and olives. Continue sautéing them for about five additional minutes.

Sprinkle the veggies with the cumin, parsley, salt, chicken bouillon, paprika, and cayenne.

Stir thoroughly and place the fish on top of the veggies.

Pour in water to cover the veggies.

Lower the heat setting and cover the pan to slowly cook until the fish is flaky (about 40 min..

Nutrition Info: Calories: 268;Protein: 42 grams; Fat: 5 grams

Niçoise-inspired Salad With Sardines

Servings: 4

Cooking Time: 15 Minutes

Ingredients:

4 eggs

12 ounces baby red potatoes (about 12 potatoes)

6 ounces green beans, halved

4 cups baby spinach leaves or mixed greens

1 bunch radishes, quartered (about 1⅓ cups)

1 cup cherry tomatoes

20 kalamata or niçoise olives (about ⅓ cup)

3 (3.75-ounce) cans skinless, boneless sardines packed in olive oil, drained

8 tablespoons Dijon Red Wine Vinaigrette

Directions:

Place the eggs in a saucepan and cover with water. Bring the water to a boil. As soon as the water starts to boil, place a lid on the pan and turn the heat off. Set a timer for minutes.

When the timer goes off, drain the hot water and run cold water over the eggs to cool. Peel the eggs when cool and cut in half.

Prick each potato a few times with a fork. Place them on a microwave-safe plate and microwave on high for 4 to 5 minutes, until the potatoes are tender. Let cool and cut in half.

Place green beans on a microwave-safe plate and microwave on high for 1½ to 2 minutes, until the beans are crisp-tender. Cool.

Place 1 egg, ½ cup of green beans, 6 potato halves, 1 cup of spinach, ⅓ cup of radishes, ¼ cup of tomatoes, olives, and 3 sardines in each of 4 containers. Pour 2 tablespoons of vinaigrette into each of 4 sauce containers.

STORAGE: Store covered containers in the refrigerator for up to 4 days.

Nutrition Info: Total calories: 450; Total fat: 32g; Saturated fat: 5g; Sodium: 6mg; Carbohydrates: 22g; Fiber: 5g; Protein: 21g

Lettuce Tomato Salad

Servings: 6

Cooking Time: 15 Minutes

Ingredients:

1 heart of Romaine lettuce, chopped

3 Roma tomatoes, diced

1 English cucumber, diced

1 small red onion, finely chopped

½ cup curly parsley, finely chopped

2 tablespoons virgin olive oil

lemon juice, ½ large lemon

1 teaspoon garlic powder

salt

pepper

Directions:

Add all Ingredients: to a large bowl.

Toss well and transfer them to containers.

Enjoy!

Nutrition Info: Calories: 68, Total Fat: 9 g, Saturated Fat: 0.8 g, Cholesterol: 0 mg, Sodium: 7 mg, Total Carbohydrate: 6 g, Dietary Fiber: 1.5 g, Total Sugars: 3.3 g, Protein: 1.3 g, Vitamin D: 0 mcg, Calcium: 18 mg, Iron: 1 mg, Potassium: 309 mg

Mediterranean Chicken Pasta Bake

Servings: 4

Cooking Time: 30 Minutes

Ingredients:

Marinade:

1½ lbs. boneless, skinless chicken thighs, cut into bite-sized
pieces*

2 garlic cloves, thinly sliced

2-3 tbsp. marinade from artichoke hearts

4 sprigs of fresh oregano, leaves stripped

Olive oil

Red wine vinegar

Pasta:

1 lb whole wheat fusilli pasta

1 red onion, thinly sliced

1 pint grape or cherry tomatoes, whole

½ cup marinated artichoke hearts, roughly chopped

½ cup white beans, rinsed + drained (I use northern white
beans)

½ cup Kalamata olives, roughly chopped

⅓ cup parsley and basil leaves, roughly chopped

2-3 handfuls of part-skim shredded mozzarella cheese

Salt, to taste

Pepper, to taste

Garnish:

Parsley

Basil leaves

Directions:

Create the chicken marinade by drain the artichoke hearts reserving the juice

In a large bowl, add the artichoke juice, garlic, chicken, and oregano leaves, drizzle with olive oil, a splash of red wine vinegar, and mix well to coat

Marinate for at least 1 hour, maximum hours

Cook the pasta in boiling salted water, drain and set aside

Preheat your oven to 42degrees F

In a casserole dish, add the sliced onions and tomatoes, toss with olive oil, salt and pepper. Then cook, stirring occasionally, until the onions are soft and the tomatoes start to burst, about 15-20 minutes

In the meantime, in a large skillet over medium heat, add 1 tsp of olive oil

Remove the chicken from the marinade, pat dry, and season with salt and pepper

Working in batches, brown the chicken on both sides, leaving slightly undercooked

Remove the casserole dish from the oven, add in the cooked pasta, browned chicken, artichoke hearts, beans, olives, and chopped herbs, stir to combine

Top with grated cheese

Bake for an additional 5-7 minutes, until the cheese is brown and bubbling

Remove from the oven and allow the dish to cool completely

Distribute among the containers, store for 2-3 days

To Serve: Reheat in the microwave for 1-2 minutes or until heated through.

Garnish with fresh herbs and serve

Nutrition Info: Calories:487;Carbs: 95g;Total Fat: 5g;Protein: 22g

Roasted Vegetable Flatbread

Servings: 12

Cooking Time: 25 Minutes

Ingredients:

16 oz pizza dough, homemade or frozen

6 oz soft goat cheese, divided

¾ cup grated Parmesan cheese divided

3 tbsp chopped fresh dill, divided

1 small red onion, sliced thinly

1 small zucchini, sliced thinly

2 small tomatoes, thinly sliced

1 small red pepper, thinly sliced into rings

Olive oil

Salt, to taste

Pepper, to taste

Directions:

Preheat the oven to 400 degrees F

Roll the dough into a large rectangle, and then place it on a piece of parchment paper sprayed with non-stick spray

Take a knife and spread half the goat cheese onto one half of the dough, then sprinkle with half the dill and half the Parmesan cheese

Carefully fold the other half of the dough on top of the cheese, spread and sprinkle the remaining parmesan and goat cheese

Layer the thinly sliced vegetables over the top

Brush the olive oil over the top of the veggies and sprinkle with salt, pepper, and the remaining dill

Bake for 22-25 minutes, until the edges are medium brown, cut in half, lengthwise

Then slice the flatbread in long 2-inch slices and allow to cool

Distribute among the containers, store for 2 days

To Serve: Reheat in the oven at 375 degrees for 5 minutes or until hot. Enjoy with a fresh salad.

Nutrition Info: Calories:170; Carbs: 21g; Total Fat: 6g; Protein: 8g

Steak Cobb Salad

Servings: 4

Cooking Time: 15 Minutes

Ingredients:

6 large eggs

2 tbsp unsalted butter

1 lb steak

2 tbsp olive oil

6 cups baby spinach

1 cup cherry tomatoes, halved

1 cup pecan halves

1/2 cup crumbled feta cheese

Kosher salt, to taste

Freshly ground black pepper, to taste

Directions:

In a large skillet over medium high heat, melt butter

Using paper towels, pat the steak dry, then drizzle with olive oil and season with salt and pepper, to taste

Once heated, add the steak to the skillet and cook, flipping once, until cooked through to desired doneness, - cook for 4 minutes per side for a medium-rare steak

Transfer the steak to a plate and allow it to cool before dicing

Place the eggs in a large saucepan and cover with cold water by 1 inch

Bring to a boil and cook for 1 minute, cover the eggs with a tight-fitting lid and remove from heat, set aside for 8-10 minutes, then drain well and allow to cool before peeling and dicing

Assemble the salad in the container by placing the spinach at the bottom of the container, top with arranged rows of steak, eggs, feta, tomatoes, and pecans

To Serve: Top with the balsamic vinaigrette, or desired dressing

Recipe Note: You can also use New York, rib-eye or filet mignon for this recipe

Nutrition Info: Calories:640;Total Fat: 51g;Total Carbs: 9.8g;Fiber: 5g;Protein: 38.8g

Grilled Lamb Chops

Servings: 4

Cooking Time: 10 Minutes

Ingredients:

4 8-ounce lamb shoulder chops

2 tablespoons Dijon mustard

2 tablespoons balsamic vinegar

1 tablespoon chopped garlic

¼ teaspoon ground black pepper

½ cup olive oil

2 tablespoons fresh basil, shredded

Directions:

Pat the lamb chops dry and arrange them in a shallow glass-baking dish.

Take a bowl and whisk in Dijon mustard, garlic, balsamic vinegar, and pepper.

Mix well to make the marinade.

Whisk oil slowly into the marinade until it is smooth.

Stir in basil.

Pour the marinade over the lamb chops, making sure to coat both sides.

Cover, refrigerate and allow the chops to marinate for anywhere from 1-4 hours.

Remove the chops from the refrigerator and leave out for 30 minutes or until room temperature.

Preheat grill to medium heat and oil grate.

Grill the lamb chops until the center reads 145 degrees F and they are nicely browned, about 5-minutes per side.

Enjoy!

Nutrition Info: Calories: 1587, Total Fat: 97.5 g, Saturated Fat: 27.6 g, Cholesterol: 600 mg, Sodium: 729 mg, Total Carbohydrate: 1.3 g, Dietary Fiber: 0.4 g, Total Sugars: 0.1 g, Protein: 176.5 g, Vitamin D: 0 mcg, Calcium: 172 mg, Iron: 15 mg, Potassium: 30 mg

Broiled Chili Calamari

Servings: 4

Cooking Time: 8 Minutes

Ingredients:

2 tablespoons extra virgin olive oil

1 teaspoon chili powder

½ teaspoon ground cumin

Zest of 1 lime

Juice of 1 lime

Dash of sea salt

1 and ½ pounds squid, cleaned and split open, with tentacles cut into ½ inch rounds

2 tablespoons cilantro, chopped

2 tablespoons red bell pepper, minced

Directions:

Take a medium bowl and stir in olive oil, chili powder, cumin, lime zest, sea salt, lime juice and pepper

Add squid and let it marinade and stir to coat, coat and let it refrigerate for 1 hour

Pre-heat your oven to broil

Arrange squid on a baking sheet, broil for 8 minutes turn once until tender

Garnish the broiled calamari with cilantro and red bell pepper

Serve and enjoy!

Meal Prep/Storage Options: Store in airtight containers in your fridge for 1-2 days.

Nutrition Info: Calories:159;Fat: 13g;Carbohydrates: 12g;Protein: 3g

Salmon With Corn Pepper Salsa

Servings: 2

Cooking Time: 12 Minutes

Ingredients:

1 garlic clove, grated

½ teaspoon mild chili powder

½ teaspoon ground coriander

¼ teaspoon ground cumin

2 limes – 1, zest and juice; 1 cut into wedges

2 teaspoons rapeseed oil

2 wild salmon fillets

1 ear of corn on the cob, husk removed

1 red onion, finely chopped

1 avocado, cored, peeled, and finely chopped

1 red pepper, deseeded and finely chopped

1 red chili, halved and deseeded

½ a pack of finely chopped coriander

Directions:

Boil the corn in water for about 6-8 minutes until tender.

Drain and cut off the kernels.

In a bowl, combine garlic, spices, 1 tablespoon of limejuice, and oil; mix well to prepare spice rub.

Coat the salmon with the rub.

Add the zest to the corn and give it a gentle stir.

Heat a frying pan over medium heat.

Add salmon and cook for about 2 minutes per side.

Serve the cooked salmon with salsa and lime wedges.

Enjoy!

Nutrition Info: Calories: 949, Total Fat: 57.4 g, Saturated Fat: 9.7 g, Cholesterol: 2mg, Sodium: 180 mg, Total Carbohydrate: 33.5 g, Dietary Fiber: 11.8 g, Total Sugars: 8.3 g, Protein: 76.8 g, Vitamin D: 0 mcg, Calcium: 100 mg, Iron: 3 mg, Potassium: 856 mg

Italian-inspired Rotisserie Chicken And Broccoli Slaw

Servings: 4 :

Cooking Time: 15 Minutes

Ingredients:

4 cups packaged broccoli slaw

1 cooked rotisserie chicken, meat removed (about 10 to 12 ounces)

1 bunch red radishes, stemmed, halved, and thickly sliced (about 1¼ cups)

1 cup sliced red onion

½ cup pitted kalamata or niçoise olives, roughly chopped

½ cup sliced pepperoncini

8 tablespoons Dijon Red Wine Vinaigrette, divided

Directions:

Place the broccoli slaw, chicken, radishes, onion, olives, and pepperoncini in a large mixing bowl. Toss to combine.

Place cups of salad in each of 4 containers. Pour 2 tablespoons of vinaigrette into each of 4 sauce containers.

STORAGE: Store covered containers in the refrigerator for up to 5 days.

Nutrition Info: Total calories: 329; Total fat: 2; Saturated fat: 4g; Sodium: 849mg; Carbohydrates: 10g; Fiber: 3g; Protein: 20g

Flatbread With Roasted Vegetables

Servings: 12

Cooking Time: 45 Minutes

Ingredients:

5 ounces goat cheese

1 thinly sliced onion

2 thinly sliced tomatoes

Olive oil

¼ teaspoon pepper

⅛ teaspoon salt

16 ounces homemade or frozen pizza dough

¾ tablespoon chopped dill, fresh is better

1 thinly sliced zucchini

1 red pepper, cup into rings

Directions:

Set your oven to 400 degrees Fahrenheit.

Set the dough on a large piece of parchment paper. Use a rolling pin to roll the dough into a large rectangle.

Spread half of the goat cheese on ½ of the pizza dough.

Sprinkle half of the dill on the other half of the dough.

Fold the dough so the half with the dill is on top of the cheese.

Spread the remaining goat cheese on the pizza dough and then sprinkle the rest of the dill over the cheese.

Layer the vegetables on top in any arrangement you like.

Drizzle olive oil on top of the vegetables.

Sprinkle salt and pepper over the olive oil.

Set the piece of parchment paper on a pizza pan or baking pan and place it in the oven.

Set the timer for 22 minutes. If the edges are not a medium brown, leave the flatbread in the oven for another couple of minutes.

Remove the pizza from the oven when it is done and cut the flatbread in half lengthwise.

Slice the flatbread into 2-inch long pieces and enjoy!

Nutrition Info: calories: 170, fats: 5 grams, carbohydrates: 20 grams, protein: 8 grams.

Seafood Paella

Servings: 4-5
Cooking Time: 40 Minutes

Ingredients:

4 small lobster tails (6-12 oz each)

Water

3 tbsp Extra Virgin Olive Oil

1 large yellow onion, chopped

2 cups Spanish rice or short grain rice, soaked in water for 15 minutes and then drained

4 garlic cloves, chopped

2 large pinches of Spanish saffron threads soaked in 1/2 cup water

1 tsp Sweet Spanish paprika

1 tsp cayenne pepper

1/2 tsp aleppo pepper flakes

Salt, to taste

2 large Roma tomatoes, finely chopped

6 oz French green beans, trimmed

1 lb prawns or large shrimp or your choice, peeled and deveined

1/4 cup chopped fresh parsley

Directions:

In a large pot, add 3 cups of water and bring it to a rolling boil

Add in the lobster tails and allow boil briefly, about 1-minutes or until pink, remove from heat

Using tongs transfer the lobster tails to a plate and Do not discard the lobster cooking water

Allow the lobster is cool, then remove the shell and cut into large chunks.

In a large deep pan or skillet over medium-high heat, add 3 tbsp olive oil

Add the chopped onions, sauté the onions for 2 minutes and then add the rice, and cook for 3 more minutes, stirring regularly

Then add in the lobster cooking water and the chopped garlic and, stir in the saffron and its soaking liquid, cayenne pepper, aleppo pepper, paprika, and salt

Gently stir in the chopped tomatoes and green beans, bring to a boil and allow the liquid slightly reduce, then cover (with lid or tightly wrapped foil) and cook over low heat for 20 minutes

Once done, uncover and spread the shrimp over the rice, push it into the rice slightly, add in a little water, if needed

Cover and cook for another 15 minutes until the shrimp turn pink

Then add in the cooked lobster chunks

Once the lobster is warmed through, remove from heat allow the dish to cool completely

Distribute among the containers, store for 2 days

To Serve: Reheat in the microwave for 1-2 minutes or until heated through. Garnish with parsley and enjoy!

Recipe Notes: Remember to soak your rice if needed to help with the cooking process

Nutrition Info: Calories:536; Carbs: 56g; Total Fat: 26g; Protein: 50g

Mediterranean Pearl Couscous

Servings: 6

Cooking Time: 10 Minutes

Ingredients:

For the Lemon Dill Vinaigrette:

1 large lemon, juice of

1/3 cup Extra virgin olive oil

1 tsp dill weed

1 tsp garlic powder

Salt and pepper

For the Israeli Couscous:

2 cups Pearl Couscous, Israeli Couscous

Extra virgin olive oil

2 cups grape tomatoes, halved

1/3 cup finely chopped red onions

1/2 English cucumber, finely chopped

15 oz can chickpeas

14 oz can good quality artichoke hearts, roughly chopped if needed

1/2 cup good pitted kalamata olives

15–20 fresh basil leaves, roughly chopped or torn; more for garnish

3 oz fresh baby mozzarella or feta cheese, optional

Water

Directions:

Make the lemon-dill vinaigrette, place the lemon juice, olive oil, dill weed, garlic powder, salt and pepper in a bowl, whisk together to combine and set aside

In a medium-sized heavy pot, heat two tbsp of olive oil

Sauté the couscous in the olive oil briefly until golden brown, then add cups of boiling water (or follow the instructed on the package), and cook according to package.

Once done, drain in a colander, set aside in a bowl and allow to cool

In a large mixing bowl, combine the extra virgin olive oil, grape tomatoes, red onions, cucumber, chickpeas, artichoke hearts, and kalamata olives

Then add in the couscous and the basil, mix together gently

Now, give the lemon-dill vinaigrette a quick whisk and add to the couscous salad, mix to combine

Taste and adjust salt, if needed

Distribute among the containers, store for 2-3 days

To Serve: Add in the mozzarella cheese, garnish with more fresh basil and enjoy!

Nutrition Info: Calories:393;Carbs: 57g;Total Fat: 13g;Protein: 13g

Potato And Tuna Salad

Servings: 4

Cooking Time: Nil

Ingredients:

1-pound baby potatoes, scrubbed, boiled

1 cup tuna chunks, drained

1 cup cherry tomatoes, halved

1 cup medium onion, thinly sliced

8 pitted black olives

2 medium hard-boiled eggs, sliced

1 head Romaine lettuce

Honey lemon mustard dressing

¼ cup olive oil

2 tablespoons lemon juice

1 tablespoon Dijon mustard

1 teaspoon dill weed, chopped

Salt as needed

Pepper as needed

Directions:

Take a small glass bowl and mix in your olive oil, honey, lemon juice, Dijon mustard and dill

Season the mix with pepper and salt

Add in the tuna, baby potatoes, cherry tomatoes, red onion, green beans, black olives and toss everything nicely

Arrange your lettuce leaves on a beautiful serving dish to make the base of your salad

Top them up with your salad mixture and place the egg slices

Drizzle it with the previously prepared Salad Dressing

Serve hot

Meal Prep/Storage Options: Store in airtight containers in your fridge for 1-2 days. Keep the fish and salad ingredients separated, mix together before serving!

Nutrition Info: Calories: 406; Fat: 22g; Carbohydrates: 28g; Protein: 26g

GREAT MEDITERRANEAN DIET RECIPES

Pumpkin, Cauliflower and Chickpea Curry

Preparation time: 5 minutes

Cooking time: 25 minutes

Servings: 4

Ingredients:

2 cup Butternut Pumpkin

1 tbsp of Oil

One sliced onion

1 Tomato diced

2 cups cauliflower Florets

1 cup Chickpeas boiled

Salt

Curry Powder

1 tsp Cumin Powder

1 tbsp Coriander powder

1 tsp Chili Powder

1/2 tsp Turmeric

Directions :

Add chopped pumpkin, onions & tomato in a pot & 1 cup of water. Now, pressure cooks it for around 6 minutes. Allow pressure to escape naturally. Blend in a blender. Add oil & cauliflower in a pot and Sauté till golden brown, 15 minutes. Add cooked chickpeas & Curry Powder & Mix Well then add Pure and bring to boil. Season with salt. Serve hot with rice.

Nutrition Info: Calories:263 kcal Fat:2 g Protein:12 g Carbs:44 g Fiber:7 g

Ratatouille

Preparation time: 20 minutes

Cooking time: 40 minutes

Servings: 8

Ingredients:

Veggies

Two zucchinis

Two eggplants

Two yellow squashes

6 Roma tomatoes

Sauce

One onion diced

Four cloves minced garlic

2 tbsp olive oil

One diced red bell pepper

One diced yellow bell pepper

Salt and pepper

28 oz crushed tomatoes

2 tbsp chopped basil

Herb seasoning

2 tbsp chopped basil

1 tsp garlic minced

2 tbsp fresh parsley Chopped

2 tsp thyme

Salt and pepper to taste

4 tbsp olive oil

Directions :

Preheat oven to 375°F.

Heat olive oil in an oven-safe pan. Sauté onion, garlic, & bell peppers for about 10 minutes. Then season with salt & pepper, add the crushed tomatoes. Mix. Remove from heat, and then add basil. Stir until smooth. Arrange sliced veggies on top of the sauce and then season with salt & pepper. In a small bowl, mix the basil, parsley, thyme, garlic, salt, pepper, & olive oil. Spoon herb seasoning on vegetables. Cover pan with foil & bake, 40 minutes. Now, Uncover, and bake for the next 20 minutes, till vegetables are softened. Serve

Nutrition Info: Calories:230 kcal Fat:11 g Protein: 5 g Carbs:32 g Fiber:8 g

Pomegranate with Orange, Parsley Gremolata and Roasted Red Onions

Preparation time: 40 minutes

Cooking time: 30 minutes

Servings: 10

Ingredients:

five tbsp olive oil

¼ cup pomegranate molasses

two tbsp vinegar red wine

one tbsp minced rosemary

two tsp coarse kosher salt

½ tsp black pepper

Five sliced red onions

Gremolata

2/3 cup pomegranate seeds

1 tbsp chopped Italian parsley

2 tsp grated orange peel

Directions :

Onions

Place the rack in the middle of the preheated oven at 425°F. Use a Line of a wide-rimmed baking sheet and put in a wide tub, whisk the first six ingredients. Add the onions; whisk gently. Add all the onions near together. A cut side down, place them on a baking sheet; Using a thin spatula, transform the onions gently. Continue to roast the onions until they are soft and thickly filled with glaze. Keep watching to avoid over-browning. Remove them from the oven.

Reheat in 350°F oven just before serving, if necessary.

Gremolata

In a tiny cup, mix the pomegranate seed with parsley and the orange peel.

Arrange onion on a plate mildly hot or at room temperature. Sprinkle with Gremolata and then serve.

Nutrition Info: Calories: 158.1kcal Fat: 40.9g Protein: 18.1 g Carbs:21.7 g Fiber: 3.6g

The easiest stir fry vegetable

Preparation time: 10 minutes

Cooking time: 5 minutes

Servings: 6

Ingredients:

1 tbsp olive oil

One sliced bell pepper red

One sliced bell pepper yellow

1 cup sugar snap peas

1 cup carrots sliced

One cup sliced mushrooms

Two cups broccoli

One cup baby corn

½ cup water chestnuts

¼ cup of soy sauce

Three minced garlic cloves

3 tbsp brown sugar

One tsp sesame oil

½ cup chicken broth

One tbsp cornstarch

Directions :

Put one tablespoon of olive oil in a large skillet over medium heat. Add red and yellow bell pepper, peas, cabbage, mushrooms, broccoli, sweet corn, and some water chestnuts.

Sauté for 2-3 minutes until the vegetables are nearly soft. In a small whisk, add soy sauce, minced garlic, brown sugar, and sesame oil. Finally, add chicken broth and cornstarch. Pour over the vegetables and boil until the sauce becomes thickened. Garnish with sliced green onions or sesame seed if needed.

Nutrition Info: Calories: 52kcal Fat:4g Protein: 5g Carbs:27 g Fiber: 4g

Mediterranean Stew on Slow Cooker

Preparation time: 30 minutes

Cooking time: 10 hours

Servings: 10

Ingredients:

One cubed squash butternut

2 cups cubed eggplant,

2 cups cubed zucchini

10 oz okra

8 oz tomato sauce

1 cup chopped onion

One Chopped tomato

sliced thin carrot, 1

vegetable broth, ½ cup

raisins, ⅓ cup

chopped garlic, one clove

ground cumin, ½ teaspoon

ground turmeric, ½ teaspoon

crushed red pepper, ¼ teaspoon

the ground cinnamon, ¼ teaspoon

paprika, ¼ teaspoon

Directions :

use a slow cooker, add butternut squash with eggplant, add
zucchini, okra, tomato sauce, cabbage, peas, carrots, broth,

raisins, and finally garlic. Season with cumin seed, turmeric, red pepper, and cinnamon. Cover and simmer for 9 to 10 hours on medium heat or until vegetables get softened.

Nutrition Info: Calories 121.9 kcal: Fat:0.5 g Protein: 3.4 g Carbs: 30.5g Fiber:7.8 g

Spinach, Bean Curry & Red Lentil

Preparation time: 25 minutes

Cooking time: 10 minutes

Servings: 4

Ingredients:

red lentils, 1 cup

tomato puree, ¼ cup

container plain yogurt, ½ (8 ounces)

garam masala, one teaspoon

ground dried turmeric, ½ teaspoon

ground cumin, ½ teaspoon

ancho Chile powder, ½ teaspoon

vegetable oil, two tablespoons

onion, chopped, 1

cloves garlic chopped, 2

ginger root piece fresh grated, 1 (1 inch)

fresh spinach, loosely packed coarsely chopped, 4 cups

chopped tomatoes, 2

chopped fresh cilantro, four sprigs

can mixed beans, 1 (15.5 ounces), rinsed and drained

Directions :

Rinse all the lentils and put them in a saucepan; add enough water to cover. Get things to a simmer. Reduce heat to medium, cover the pot and boil for 20 minutes over medium heat. In a bowl, combine the purée of tomatoes and the yogurt. Season with some garam masala, then add turmeric and cumin; finally, mix some chili powder. Stir until creamy. Heat oil over low heat. Stir in the onion, garlic, and 1" piece of ginger; simmer until the onion starts to brown. Now Stir in spinach; boil until dark green colored and wilt. Gradually stir in a combination of yogurt. Mix with tomatoes and cilantro. Stir the lentils and beans in the mixture until well balanced. Heat through maybe five minutes.

Nutrition Info: Calories: 328kcal Fat:8.3 g Protein:18 g Carbs:51.9 g Fiber:15.4 g

Giant stuffed capsicum

Preparation time:15 minutes

Cooking time: 15 minutes

Servings: 5

Ingredients:

large capsicum/peppers, 5

olive oil, one tablespoon

chopped onion, 1

garlic cloves, minced, 3

lean ground beef, 350 g (12oz)

tomato paste, 1/4 cup

chicken broth/stock, 1/4 cups (315 ml)

grain rice, 1/2 cup uncooked

corn kernels, 1 cup

finely sliced green onions, 1 cup,

shredded mozzarella, 1 1/2 cups (150g)

water, 1/2 cup (125 ml)

Mexican spices

cayenne pepper, 1/2 teaspoon

dried oregano, one tablespoon

cumin, two teaspoons

coriander, two teaspoons

onion powder, 1.5 teaspoons

salt 3/4 teaspoon

Directions :

Preheat the oven to 170C/350F.

Hollow peppers. Using a tiny knife, slit the top of capsicum at 45 °angle. Drop empty seeds from the end. in case the capsicum bottoms are not quite straight, cut them to lie flat. (Be sure to break out in little piece so that you don't inadvertently cut a hole just in the bottom)

Place the capsicums over the baking dish and suits them snugly.

Filling .Heat oil in a broad skillet over medium heat; Add the onion and garlic, then roast for 2 minutes.

Attach beef and fry, split it while you move, before it's all modified from pink to blue.

Add the herbs, stir. Finally, add some tomato paste and simmer for 1 minute.

Add the barley, the maize, and the chicken broth. Now Bring to a boil, put the lid on and reduce the heat to low heat. Cook for about 13-15 minutes before the rice has been cooked in the mixture; they should still be very loose at this point, not dense and stodgy (see video).

Stir the green onion. Fill & back. Put half of the filling in the packed capsicums.

Nutrition Info: Calories: 387kcal Fat: 15g Protein: 27 g Carbs:36 g Fiber:5 g

Teriyaki Sesame Vegetables

Preparation time: 15 minutes

Cooking time: 15 minutes

Servings: 4

Ingredients:

Tempeh,1 package / 8 ounce

medium heads broccoli, 2

green, red, and yellow bell peppers, 3

freshly minced ginger root, one teaspoon

small green onions, 5

sesame oil, 1 1/2 tablespoons

Directions :

Break the tempeh into the shape of rectangles. Break the broccoli into the shape of bulbs. Break the peppers into broad parts. Peel and cut the ginger. Slice fine pieces of the green onion. Use a large skillet, melt one tablespoon of sesame oil over low heat. Add the tempeh into a single sheet, sprinkle few pinches of kosher salt, and 3 to 4 minutes per side until you get them lightly browned. Remove it from the jar. Add half a tablespoon of sesame oil in the same skillet. Now add the broccoli; also add a couple of pinches of kosher salt. Then slowly cook while stirring continuously, for 1 minute. Finally, add half a cup of water and proceed to Sautee; add some ginger and peppers with green onion and add another pinch of salt until the water boils out about 2 minutes). Sauté until all the vegetables are soft, around 4 to 5 minutes.

Switch the heat off. Add all the tempeh with teriyaki sauce and mix until it is filled with sauce. Now taste and apply, if necessary, a pinch of salt. Garnish with some sesame seed and serve it with the rice

Nutrition Info: Calories: 385 kcal Fat:9 g Protein:17.6 g Carbs:58.8 g Fiber:8.49 g

Vegetarian Cannelloni

Preparation time:15 minutes
Cooking time: 45 minutes
Servings:6

Ingredients:

taco mixed beans, 395 g tin
olive oil, one tablespoon
chopped and peeled onion, 1
chopped red pepper, 1
chopped yellow pepper, 1
passata 500g carton, with garlic and herbs
cannelloni, 12 tubes
grated Cheddar mature, 200g
mixed leaves, to serve

Directions :

Preheat an oven to 150°C or 190°C, and fan 170°C.

Use a bowl and place the beans, now mash until they have been coarsely smashed. Set it back.

Heat some oil in a medium frying pan. Now add the onion and cook on low heat for 3 minutes. Switch off the fire, add peppers, and then stir-fry for 4-5 minutes. Remove from flame and let it cool slightly. Apply the spice mixture into the beans finally stir well. Set it back.

Place one-third of the passata using a 20 by 30cm baking dish and simply set aside.

Fill all the cannelloni tubes using pepper and bean mixture with the help of a teaspoon. Organize in the bowl, then spill over all the remaining passata, then sprinkle with grated cheese. Now bake for 45 minutes or until golden brown and bubbly. Serve hot

Nutrition Info: Calories: 711 kcal Fat:47 g Protein:30 g Carbs:44 g Fiber:5 g

Corn and Zucchini Fritters

Preparation time: 15 minutes

Cooking time: 4 minutes

Servings: 12

Ingredients:

all-purpose flour,2 cups

baking powder, one tablespoon

cumin, ½ teaspoon

sugar, ½ cup

salt, ½ teaspoon

eggs, beaten, 2

milk, 1 cup

melted butter, ¼ cup

grated zucchini, 2 cups

fresh corn, 1 ½ cups

Cheddar cheese finely shredded, 1 cup

oil for frying

Directions :

In a big cup, mix flour and baking powder add cumin, sugar with salt and pepper.

In a shallow cup, mix the eggs and milk with butter together.

Whisk the wet ingredients with the dry ingredients. Finally, Stir in courgette, corn, and cheese; blend well.

Heat some oil in a steel skillet over low heat. Add the spoonful of the batter to the hot liquid. Fry until brown. Turn the tongs once. Drop on the paper towels.

Nutrition Info: Calories:143 kcal Fat: 8g Protein: 3.6g Carbs:15 g Fiber: 0.7 g

Grilled Aubergine Panini

Preparation time:10 minutes

Cooking time:25 minutes

Servings:4

Ingredients:

Mayonnaise reduced-fat, two tablespoons

Fresh basil sliced, two tablespoons

Extra-virgin olive oil, separated, two tablespoons

Eggplant slices, 8 ounces 8 1/2-inch

Garlic salt ½ teaspoon

Whole-grain country bread, eight slices

Fresh mozzarella cheese, 8 ounces 8 thin slices

Roasted red peppers sliced jarred, ⅓ cup

Red onion, four pieces four thin slices

Directions :

Preheat grill to about medium-high flame. In a shallow tub, mix mayonnaise and basil. Using one tablespoon of the oil, gently brush both the sides of the eggplant and then sprinkle each piece with garlic salt. Coat one side of every piece of bread using the residual one tablespoon of the oil.

Grill the eggplant now for about 6 minutes, turning its side with the spatula, covering with the cheese, and then proceeding to grill till the cheese gets melted. The eggplant is soft, around 4 minutes longer. Cook the bread upon this grill for about 1 to 2 minutes each foot.

To produce sandwiches: scatter the mayonnaise basil over four pieces of bread. Cover with cheesy eggplant, red pepper, onion, and the remaining pieces of bread. Break it in half, then serve hot.

Nutrition Info: Calories: 354 kcal Fat:17.1 g Protein:15 g Carbs:34.5 g Fiber: 6.7 g

Roasted Vegetable Frittata

Preparation time:30 minutes

Cooking time:55 minutes

Servings: 4

Ingredients:

Orange sweet potato, skinned, cut into pieces (3cm), 350g

Red capsicum, cut into pieces (3cm), 1

Red onions, cut into wedges, 2

Zucchini, cut into pieces (3cm), 2

Olive oil as cooking spray

Eggs 6

Skim milk 1/3 cup

Baby rocket 100g

Parmesan cheese, shaved, 20g

Walnuts, roughly sliced, 1/4 cup

Balsamic vinegar, one tablespoon

Directions :

Preheat the oven to about 220°C. Oiled e a 6cm in-depth, 20cm wide, 8-cup square oven-safe bowl. Line up a broad roasting pan with the baking paper. Put the sweet potatoes, capsicum, onions with zucchini in the tub. Spray the gasoline. Place in a single thin layer and toast for about 30 minutes until it becomes golden and soft.

Spread the vegetables on the base of the prepared bowl. Reduce oven to a temperature of 190°C. Mix the eggs, the milk as well as the pepper together in a cup. Pour the egg mixture over the vegetables, shake the dish gently to allow the egg to disperse to the base. Bake the frittata for about 25 minutes or until the top is golden and the middle is set. Put aside for ten minutes. Break the mixture into 4 bits.

Place the rocket, the parmesan, and the walnuts in a dish. Toss to mix it. Divide the salad and the frittata onto the serving dishes. Drop one teaspoon of vinegar into each salad. Now serve it

Nutrition Info: Calories:1215 kcal Fat:15.6 g Protein:16.8 g Carbs:198 g Fiber:4.2 g

Pita Pockets

Preparation time: 3 hours

Cooking time: 10 minutes

Servings: 6

Ingredients:

Wheat Flour, 2 cups

Maida (All-purpose flour), two tablespoons

Active dry yeast, one packet

Sugar, one teaspoon

Milk or warm water, 3/4 – 1 cup

Oil, one tablespoon

Salt, as per taste

Directions :

Put all the products together. Preheat the oven to 400 degrees F. Dissolve the yeast with sugar in the warm milk or water and leave to stand for about 2-3 minutes till it becomes foamy. Once the yeast is activated (foamy and bubbly), continue with the recipe. In case the yeast ceases to do so, kindly discard and start anew. When the yeast has sprouted, mix all the ingredients inside a tub, add the yeast with oil then knead the dough. Wrap the dough now with a moist cloth, then set aside for about 2-3 hours. The dough would almost become double in size. Divide the dough into similar balls.

Roll these in thick rings. Put the rolled dough over the baking sheet, then bake inside the oven for about 7-10 minutes till it becomes brown from the tip.

You'll see them buffing up shortly. All puffed up. Take them out from the oven, then let them cool down. Now serve the Pita bread pockets.

Nutrition Info: Calories:198 kcal Fat:4 g Protein:5 g Carbs:35 g Fiber:1 g

Chicken Guacamole Wraps

Preparation time:5 minutes

Cooking time:5 minutes

Servings: 4

Ingredients:

Fresh lime juice, two tablespoons

Salt, ¼ teaspoon

Peeled avocado, one ripe

Seeded plum tomato chopped, ½ cup

Lettuce leaves, four green leaf

Flour tortillas (fat-free), 4 (8-inch)

Grilled Lemon-Herb Chicken, 2 cups (about 8 ounces)

Directions :

Put three ingredients first in a mixing saucepan; crush with a fork till smooth. Stir in the tomatoes. Put one lettuce leaf around each tortilla; scatter around 1/4 cup of avocado paste over each lettuce leaf. Cover each portion with 1/2 cup of Roasted Lemon-Herb Chicken. Now roll-up. Cover either in foil or parchment, then chill

Nutrition Info: Calories: 300 kcal Fat:10.98 g Protein:21.1 g Carbs:30.2 g Fiber:4.1 g

Italian Eggplant Salad

Preparation time: minutes

Cooking time: minutes

Servings:4

Ingredients:

3 cups Cubed eggplant

2 tbsp White wine vinegar

One clove Chopped garlic

One Chopped onion

1/2 teaspoon oregano

3 tsp Olive oil

1/4 teaspoon black pepper

One Chopped tomato

Directions : Boil water in a saucepan. Add eggplant to boiling water in a saucepan.

Add eggplant in the boiling water and cook until tender (for about 10 minutes)

Drain the water and place onion and eggplant in a glass dish. Mix vinegar, pepper, and garlic together. Pour the mixture over eggplant and onion. Toss the mixture, eggplant, and onion together. Before serving, stir in oil.

Nutrition Info: Calories: 94.6 kcal Fat: 3.8 g Protein: 2.4 g Carbs: 15.5 g Fiber: 7.8 g

Cauliflower in Mustard Sauce

Preparation time: 10 minutes

Cooking time: 90 minutes

Servings: 4

Ingredients:

1 tsp Honey

2 tsp Dijon mustard

1 ½ tbsp White-wine vinegar

Dash black pepper

1 tbsp Olive oil

2 cups cauliflower flowerets

Directions :

Mix the mustard and honey in a bowl. Add olive oil and vinegar to the bowl; Whisk Season with black pepper. Set the bowl aside. Boil water in a saucepan and add cauliflower to it. Cook until tender.

Drain the cauliflower well and add it to the mixture prepared earlier; Toss.

Give 30-45 minutes for the salad to cool down. Serve.

Nutrition Info: Calories: 343 kcal Fat: 23 g Protein: 8 g Carbs: 30 g Fiber: 7 g

Pineapple Coleslaw

Preparation time: 5 minutes

Cooking time: 0 minute

Servings: 4

Ingredients:

2 cups shredded Cabbage

1/4 cup Miracle Whip

8 oz crushed pineapples

Pepper to taste

1/4 cup chopped onion

Directions :

Take a bowl. Add all the ingredients together; mix well.

Chill for 1 hour (at least). Serve

Nutrition Info: Calories: 160 kcal Fat: 13 g Protein: 1 g Carbs: 9 g Fiber: 1 g

Basil Oil

Preparation time: 10 minutes

Cooking time: 10 minutes

Servings: 16

Ingredients:

1 cup Olive oil

1.5 cups Basil leaves

Directions :

Drain and Rinse the basil leaves. Allow them to dry by patting them with a towel.

Add and Whirl basil leaves and olive oil in a blender or food processor (until leaves are finely chopped). Do not puree.

Take a 1 to 1 1/2-quart pan. Pour the mixture into the pan, heated medium.

Stir occasionally for 3-4 minutes (look for oil bubbles to gather around pan sides and when the thermometer reaches 165 degrees, remove the pan from the stove). To kill bacteria, make sure the oil is heated to the mentioned temperature. Let the mixture cool (minimum one hour).

Take a fine wire strainer and line it with two layers of cheesecloth. Set the strainer over a small bowl. Pour the earlier prepared oil mixture into the strainer.

Let the oil passes through. Afterward, keep gently pressing the basil to the remaining oil.

Discard the leftover basil in the strainer.

For three months, store the oil in an airtight container (refrigerate). Don't worry if the olive oil solidifies when chilled. It will quickly liquefy when you bring it back to room temperature. (You can serve the oil right-away as well)

Nutrition Info: Calories: 82 kcal Fat: 9 g Protein: 0.5 g Carbs: 0.5 g Fiber: 0.5 g

Blasted Brussel Sprouts

Preparation time: 8 minutes

Cooking time: 20 minutes

Servings: 2-3

Ingredients:

3 tbsp Grated Parmesan Cheese

2 cups Brussels Sprouts

1/4 cup Fruit or herb-flavored vinegar

2 tbsp Olive oil

Directions :

Preheat oven at 450 degrees.

Firstly, clean the old leaves off. Cut all the larger sprouts in half. Leave all the smaller sprouts whole. Add olive oil; toss. Put an oiled baking sheet (lightly oiled) on.

Roast for a while (about 10 minutes) until the sprouts are tender enough to be pierced using a fork. Take out of the oven. Sprinkle with and Parmesan cheese and fruit vinegar.

Nutrition Info: Calories: 116 kcal Fat: 7 g Protein: 4 g Carbs: 12 g Fiber: 4 g

Roasted Tomatillo Salsa

Preparation time: 10 minutes

Cooking time: 10 minutes

Servings: 8

Ingredients:

1 lb Tomatillos

One Head garlic

¼ cup Water

One bunch Cilantro

Three Jalapenos

Lime juice to taste

Directions :

Take tomatillos, cut them in half. Take an Oil baking sheet. Spread tomatillos, jalapenos, and garlic, on it. Coat with oil; toss. Turn the tomatillos brown (for about 10-15 minutes). Remove from heat (oven).

Take a food processor, blend all the ingredients, including tomatillos (until everything is smooth). Serve with corn chips over burritos, tacos, or enchiladasors.

Nutrition Info: Calories: 31 kcal Fat: 0 g Protein: 2 g Carbs: 7 g Fiber: 1 g

Pico de Gallo

Preparation time: 15 minutes

Cooking time: 0 minute

Servings: 2-3

Ingredients:

Three chopped bell Peppers

One cup Jicama

Salt to taste

5 Garlic cloves

1 tbsp Sugar

½ chopped Purple onion

To taste Lime Juice

Directions :

Take a Food processor; Add all ingredients in it. Pulse and enjoy your salsa!

Nutrition Info: Calories: 33 kcal Fat: 0.2 g Protein: 0.7 g Carbs: 7.4 g Fiber: 1.9 g

Beans and Ham

Preparation time: 10 minutes

Cooking time: 50 minutes

Servings: 6

Ingredients:

1/2 cup ham

One cup White rice

One cup lima beans

4 Garlic cloves

1.5 cups diced Onion

2 tbsp Cider vinegar

1 tbsp Honey

3 tbsp Oil

Two Jalapeno peppers

½ tsp Smoked paprika

32 oz Chicken broth

½ tsp Ground pepper

¼ tsp Salt

Directions :

Add rice and beans in a pressure cooker with low sodium chicken broth and 2 cups water. Cook as per instructions of the pressure cooker (about 45 minutes for un-soaked and dry beans. Then 20 minutes at pressure. Then go for natural release).

Set the beans aside. Chop garlic and onions and sauté in oil. Set Aside. Take a small bowl; combine the honey, vinegar, salt, paprika, jalapenos, and pepper to make your seasoning.
Add the seasoning mix, onion, and garlic to the rice and beans, along with the ham. Mix and Serve!

Nutrition Info: Calories: 200 kcal Fat: 8.5 g Protein: 6.8 g Carbs: 25 g Fiber: 3.1 g

Sweet Korean Lentils

Preparation time: 5 minutes

Cooking time: 15 minutes

Servings: 4

Ingredients:

For Sauce:

2 cups Water

2 tbsp Brown sugar

¼ cup Coconut amino's

Two chopped Garlic cloves

½ tsp Crushed red pepper

One minced Ginger

1 tsp Sesame oil

For Lentils

1 tbsp Olive oil

½ chopped Yellow onion

One cup red lentil

Two sliced Green onions

Directions :

Take a jar or a measuring cup (large). Mix all the (sauce) ingredients.

Take oil in a large pot, and heat (medium-high heat).Now add the onion and sauté (about 3-5 minutes). Wait until the onion begins to brown and becomes soft Add the sauce and lentils. Gently boil. Bring to a gentle boil.

Simmer, cover, and cook (about 8-10 minutes).Wait until the lentils are tender and the liquid is absorbed (mostly). Serve by spooning the lentils in four servings. You can also garnish them with green onions (optional).

Nutrition Info: Calories: 513 kcal Fat: 9 g Protein: 20 g Carbs: 93 g Fiber: 13 g +

Chickpea Sunflower Sandwich

Preparation time: 20 minutes

Cooking time: 0 minute

Servings: 4

Ingredients:

Garlic Herb Sauce

1 tbsp Lemon juice

¼ cup Prepared hummus

2 tbsp dill

Water as needed

Two minced Garlic cloves

Chickpea Sunflower Sandwich

1 tbsp Maple syrup

¼ cup Sunflower seeds roasted

15 oz chickpeas

3 tbsp Mayonnaise

1/2 tsp Dijon or spicy mustard

Pepper to taste

¼ chopped Red onion

Eight slices of wheat bread

2 tbsp dill

Optional Toppings

Lettuce

Sliced avocado

Tomato

Onion

Directions :

To prepare the sauce (garlic herb): mix minced garlic, dill, lemon, and hummus in a bowl. Now set aside. In another bowl, mash the chickpeas roughly. To add texture, leave some in large chunks. Then add vegan mayo or tahini, sunflower seeds, maple syrup, mustard, chopped dill, pepper, and red onion. Mix them. Toast bread in vegan oil or butter (optional). Take four slices of bread. Scoop your sunflower seed filling and chickpeas on them. Add the garlic herb sauce along with your optional toppings. Top with the more four slices of bread to form a sandwich.

Nutrition Info: Calories: 532 kcal Fat: 30 g Protein: 17 g Carbs: 52 g Fiber: 14 g

Balsamic Vinaigrette

Preparation time: 4 minutes

Cooking time: 0 minute

Servings: 4

Ingredients:

¼ cup Balsamic vinegar

1 tbsp Dijon mustard

2 tbsp Honey

¾ cup Canola Oil

One Garlic clove

½ tsp black pepper

1 tsp Poppyseed

Directions :

Take a food processor and blend all ingredients in it for 3-4 minutes, thoroughly emulsified. (You can also take a jar and shake all the ingredients vigorously in it, as an alternative)

Nutrition Info: Calories: 126 kcal Fat: 8.3 g Protein: 1 g Carbs: 13 g Fiber: 0.5 g

Easy Chia Seed Pudding

Preparation time: 5 minutes

Cooking time: 0 minute

Servings: 4

Ingredients:

½ cup Chia Seeds

1.5 cup of rice milk

1 tsp Vanilla Extract

¼ tsp Cinnamon

¼ cup Maple Syrup

Directions :

Take a bowl or a mason jar, add the chia seeds, maple syrup, vanilla, rice milk, and cinnamon. Mix well! Make sure chia seeds do not stick to container sides. Cover the mixture and refrigerate (at least 4 hours or even overnight). You can also add fruit (optional) before serving.

Nutrition Info: Calories: 164 kcal Fat: 11.8 g Protein: 3.3 g Carbs: 12.4 g Fiber: 6.9 g

Herb Pesto

Preparation time: 5 minutes

Cooking time: 0 minute

Servings: 4-5

Ingredients:

½ cup Parsley leaves

1 cup basil leaves

2 Garlic cloves

½ cup Oregano leaves

2 tbsp lemon juice

¼ cup Olive oil

Directions :

Put the garlic, basil, oregano, and parsley in a food processor; pulse (for 3 minutes until finely chopped). Form a thick paste by Drizzling the olive oil on the pesto. Scrape down the sides as well.

Add the pulse and lemon juice; Blend. Take a sealed container and store the pesto in it; Refrigerate (for one week).

Nutrition Info: Calories: 22 kcal Fat: 2 g Protein: 0 g Carbs: 0 g Fiber: 10 g

Smoothie Bowl

Preparation time: 4 minutes

Cooking time: 0 minute

Servings: 1

Ingredients:

1 tbsp shredded coconut

¾ cup blueberries

1 tsp Honey

½ sliced banana

3 tbsp plain coconut milk

1 tbsp Blueberries

½ cup of Organic and Frozen strawberries

½ cup Water

Directions :

Combine all the smoothie bowl ingredients (except coconut and fresh berries) in a high-speed blender. Allow all the ingredients to be like a creamy sorbet; blend.

Pour the mixture into a bowl Garnish the smoothie with coconut and fresh berries. Eat!

Nutrition Info: Calories: 224 kcal Fat: 4 g Protein: 2 g Carbs: 51 g Fiber: 9 g

Irish Colcannon

Preparation time: 5 minutes

Cooking time: 30 minutes

Servings: 6

Ingredients:

85 g Russet potato

Three Parsnips

1.5 cup Green peas

1 cup Green cabbage

One diced Onion

1 cup chopped Kale

3 tbsp Olive oil

Black pepper to taste

Two minced Garlic cloves

Sea salt

Directions :

Place potato and parsnips in a pot of water (large) and bring the ingredients to a boil. Cook until tender (over high heat) for about fifteen minutes. Use a sieve to remove the cooked vegetables. Do not drain the remaining cooking liquid left in the pot; reserve for later.

Take a shallow bowl, and with 1/3 cup of the cooking liquid and 2 tbsp. Of the olive oil, mash the vegetables in it. Keep adding as much cooking liquid as required to remove the lumps. You can also use a hand blender. Layout mashed parsnip mixture on a foil-covered plate.

Now, add chopped kale and shredded cabbage to the parsnip water. Cook until the cabbage is just slack (for a few minutes). For this step, drain the kale and cabbage thoroughly and return them to the pot. Cover. Take a skillet (large) and heat 1 tbsp of olive oil in it using medium heat. Add and cook the chopped garlic and onion until it softens.

Further, also add the cooked garlic and onions to the pot with the greens and cabbage. Now also add the peas. In the middle of an empty serving bowl, place the parsnip and potato mash. Add and mix the cooked vegetables in. Season with salt and pepper. Serve! (As lunch or as a side dish).

Nutrition Info: Calories: 160 kcal Fat: 7 g Protein: 4 g Carbs: 21 g Fiber: 5 g

Vegan Banana Bread

Preparation time: 5 minutes

Cooking time: 60 minutes

Servings: 12

Ingredients:

1/3 cup Vegetable oil

2 tbsp Agave nectar

1/8 tsp Salt

1.5 cup Whole wheat flour

½ cup Applesauce

1 tsp Baking soda

Four Bananas

1.5 tsp Vanilla extract

½ Sugar

4 tbsp Flax seeds

Directions :

Preheat the oven to 350°F.

Firstly, peel the bananas and then mash the peeled bananas with a fork. Place the mashed bananas in a mixing bowl. Now, take a wooden spoon and mix the mashed bananas with vegetable oil using it.

Add sugar, applesauce, salt, vanilla, baking soda, agave nectar, and ground flaxseeds in the bowl; stir. Add flour and Stir thoroughly. Pour the mixture into a 9 x 5 x 3-inch loaf pan (greased). Bake for a good 50-60 minutes, until the (top) springs back become slightly depressed. Cool and serve!

Nutrition Info: Calories: 200 kcal Fat: 7 g Protein: 3 g Carbs: 33 g Fiber: 3 g

Vegetable Broth

Preparation time: 10 minutes
Cooking time: 60 minutes
Servings: 2

Ingredients:

2 cups Sliced celery stalks
2 tbsp Olive oil
Four chopped carrots
Two chopped onions
½ tsp Dried thyme
Eight cups Water
¼ cup Italian parsley
Two Bay leaves
4 Garlic cloves
1 tsp Black peppercorns

Directions :

Take a large saucepan, and heat oil in it over medium heat. Add garlic, celery, carrots, and onions. Cook and stir (occasionally) for about 5 minutes. Add peppercorns, water, thyme, parsley, and bay leaves. Set the heat to high now. Bring it to a boil. Now stir again while also reducing heat to medium-low.

Let the mixture simmer for about an hour, uncovered. Take a fine-mesh strainer and place it over a large pot. Pour all contents into the strainer. Reserve the broth while discarding the solids.

Nutrition Info: Calories: 42 kcal Fat: 1.6 g Protein: 2.4 g Carbs: 5.2 g Fiber: 2.1 g

Festive Cranberry Stuffing

Preparation time: 5 minutes

Cooking time: 30 minutes

Servings: 4

Ingredients:

1 cup diced tart apples

¼ tsp Poultry seasoning

3 cups Soft bread

2 tbsp butter

¼ cup Apple juice

¼ cup chopped celery

½ cup diced cranberries

Directions :

Preheat the oven to 350°F. Take a large bowl. In it, combine all ingredients; toss and mix.

Take a casserole dish (lightly greased). Place the mixture in it and Bake for 30 minutes.

Nutrition Info: Calories: 151 kcal Fat: 7 g Protein: 3 g Carbs: 20 g Fiber: 2 g

Simple Puerto Rican Sofrito

Preparation time: 5 minutes

Cooking time: 0 minute

Servings: 24

Ingredients:

One chopped Spanish onion

1 tsp salt

Five Stemmed aji dulce peppers

One bunch Cilantro

1 Chopped green pepper

10 Garlic cloves

Directions :

Wash all the ingredients thoroughly before using. Take a blender. Add onions first, and then add all the other ingredients (in small batches). To use within a week, you will be required to refrigerate a portion of your sofrito (in an airtight container. To use within four months or so, freeze in in an ice cube tray or small containers. It is not required to thaw before cooking.

Add 2 tbsp. Of sofrito if and whenever you make rice, soups, beans, and stews!

Nutrition Info: Calories: 10 kcal Fat: 0 g Protein: 0 g Carbs: 2 g Fiber: 0 g

Vegetable Curry

Preparation time: 30 minutes

Cooking time: 30 minutes

Servings: 5

Ingredients:

1 tsp Fennel seeds

1 tsp Cumin seeds

1 tbsp Coconut oil

Two cups Basmati rice

1 tsp Coriander seeds

1 tsp Mustard seeds

1 tsp Hot chili flakes

¼ tsp Black peppercorns

One grated ginger

One chopped Onion

1 tsp Turmeric

One chopped Carrot

6 oz Coconut milk

1.5 cups chopped Cauliflower

One cup Green peas

Directions :

Take a cast-iron skillet, and add dry spices to it. Heat (low-medium heat) for 2 minutes.

Cook the rice while the spices are heating up. (As per the directions on the package).

Add coconut oil and sauté for about 2-3 minutes (low-medium heat). Heat until the spices start popping and turn brownish.

Add ginger, hot chili flakes, and turmeric. Cook (low-medium heat) until aromatic for about six minutes.

Remove from heat make a paste of the cooked spices by blending them with the onion.

Take a separate pan, and heat the coconut milk in it until it starts to bubble up. Add the spice paste; whisk.

Add all the vegetables and for 10 minutes, let them simmer until tender.

Serve over rice (as per need) and enjoy!

Nutrition Info: Calories: 318 kcal Fat: 20 g Protein: 6 g Carbs: 30 g Fiber: 6 g

Broccoli, Lemon, and Almond Butter

Preparation time: 5 minutes

Cooking time: 10 minutes

Servings: 4

Ingredients:

One fresh broccoli florets

¼ cup melted butter

2 tbsp lemon juice

1 tsp lemon zest

¼ cup slivered almonds

Directions : Boil the broccoli till it gets tender, about 4 to 8 minutes, and then Drain. Melt the butter in a small saucepan over medium-low heat. Then remove from the heat. Stir in lemon zest, lemon juice & almonds. Pour it on hot broccoli Serve.

Nutrition Info: Calories:170 kcal Fat:15.7 g Protein:3.7 g Carbs:7 g Fiber:2.7 g

Lentils Stuffed Butternut

Preparation time:15 minutes

Cooking time: 60 minutes

Servings: 2

Ingredients:

For the squash

One butternut squash

25g Butter

Pinch of black pepper

Pinch of salt

For the stuffing

2 tsp olive oil

One clove of garlic crushed

One red onion sliced

1-inch ginger piece grated

1/2 tsp cinnamon ground

1/2 tsp cumin seeds

1/2 tsp paprika

50g Sultanas

1 cup green lentils

1 cup spinach chopped

Directions Preheat oven to 200°C.

Place squash halves in an ovenproof dish, oil it & season with salt & fresh black pepper. Roast for around 40 mins till cooked.

Heating oil in the frying pan, add garlic & red onion, then cook, occasionally stir about 5 mins. Add all other ingredients & cook for 10 minutes on low heat till the flavors are combined. Stir frequently. Add spinach & cook for 3 to 4 mins. Place stuffing mixture on the top of roasted squash, return to the oven, 10-15 minutes. Serve immediately with pan juices to be spooned over.

Nutrition Info: Calories: 354kcal Fat: g Protein: g Carbs: g Fiber: g

Green Curry Shrimp & Green Beans

Preparation time: 15 minutes

Cooking time: 30 minutes

Servings: 4

Ingredients:

Curry Paste

1 tbsp ginger minced

One onion peeled

Six cloves peeled garlic

Two jalapeños

1/2 cup cilantro & basil

1 tbsp fish sauce

1 tbsp lime juice

1 tbsp brown sugar

Shrimp & Green Beans

12 ounces trimmed green beans

16 oz of rice noodles

2 tsp cooking oil

4 cup chicken stock

15 oz coconut milk

1-pound shrimp peeled

Salt & pepper

Garnish

Ten mint torn leaves

1/2 lime juice

1/3 cup peanuts crushed

Directions: Combine all ingredients for curry paste in food processor & pulse till combined. Set it aside. Boil green beans & cook for 1 to 3 minutes till bright green & tender-crisp. Now drain & run under cold water. Transfer to a bowl & set aside. In an additional pot, cook noodles. Drain & rinse & set aside. Heat cooking oil. Add green curry paste & cook, 1-2 minutes.
Add chicken stock & stir. Bring to boil & taste & season with salt & pepper. Add coconut milk & cook, 5 minutes. Turn pot to heat. Add shrimp & cook, 5-6 minutes' till cooked. Add green beans & cook, 1 to 2 minutes. Taste & season. Combine lime juice, cashews, & mint leaves. Season with a pinch of salt. Garnish with mint leaves & cashews & serve with lime rounds.
Serve.

Nutrition Info: Calories: 680 kcal Fat:35 g Protein:37 g Carbs:59 g Fiber:5 g

www.ingramcontent.com/pod-product-compliance
Lightning Source LLC
Chambersburg PA
CBHW050752030426
42336CB00012B/1784